Hep C Treatment

Discover How to Treat and Cure Your Hepatitis C (Hep C)

by Wendy Johanson

Table of Contents

Introduction 1

Chapter 1: Understanding Hepatitis C 7

Chapter 2: Cause and Symptoms of Hepatitis C 13

Chapter 3: How to Treat Hepatitis C 17

Chapter 4: Home Prevention and Treatment 23

Chapter 5: Complementary Treatments for Hepatitis C 31

Chapter 6: Complications of Hepatitis C 41

Chapter 7: Valuable Pointers about Hepatitis C 47

Conclusion 53

Introduction

There is no one singular way of eradicating a Hepatitis C infection. Rather, it takes a combination of treatment methods and alternative therapies to get rid of Hep C and prevent the virus from multiplying and the inflammation in the body from spreading.

Taking medication is just a small part of the solution. Of course, it's critical for the treatment medications to be used properly to ensure their effectiveness. Also, it's important to consider their contra-indications and harmful side effects. As with any medication, you'll need to be aware of what these medications are and understand their actions in your body.

But as I mentioned, getting rid of the Hep C infection will involve a lot more than just taking medication. There are also factors in your lifestyle that can aide in the elimination of the virus from your system. If you or a loved one is infected with the Hepatitis C virus, the treatment combinations presented in this book can help cure the symptoms of the condition. I'm going to tell you all about the Hep C therapeutic drugs, the side effects of these drugs, other alternative methods of treatment — including home treatment methods and suggested lifestyle changes — as well as specific techniques on how to prevent the spread of Hep C to other members of your family.

© Copyright 2015 by Miafn LLC - All rights reserved.

This document is geared towards providing reliable information in regards to the topic and issue covered. The publication is sold with the idea that the publisher is not required to render accounting, officially permitted, or otherwise, qualified services. If advice is necessary, legal or professional, a practiced individual in the profession should be ordered.

- From a Declaration of Principles which was accepted and approved equally by a Committee of the American Bar Association and a Committee of Publishers and Associations.

In no way is it legal to reproduce, duplicate, or transmit any part of this document in either electronic means or in printed format. Recording of this publication is strictly prohibited and any storage of this document is not allowed unless with written permission from the publisher. All rights reserved.

The information provided herein is stated to be truthful and consistent, in that any liability, in terms of inattention or otherwise, by any usage or abuse of any policies, processes, or directions contained within is solely and completely the responsibility of the recipient reader. Under no circumstances will any legal responsibility or blame be held against the publisher for any reparation, damages, or monetary loss due to the information herein, either directly or indirectly.

Respective authors own all copyrights not held by the publisher.

The information herein is offered for informational purposes solely, and is universal as so. The presentation of the information is without contract or any type of guarantee assurance.

The trademarks that are used are without any consent, and the publication of the trademark is without permission or backing by the trademark owner. All trademarks and brands within this book are for clarifying purposes only and are the owned by the owners themselves, not affiliated with this document.

Chapter 1: Understanding Hepatitis C

Hepatitis C is one of the types of Hepatitis conditions that can affect the liver. Hepatitis is the inflammation of the liver that is caused by any of these types of viruses A, B, C, D and E. Each of these viruses has specific properties that can identify them from one another. Proper identification is needed so that appropriate treatment can be instituted.

Types of viral Hepatitis

Hepatitis A

This is the most common type of Hepatitis. It is also called "infectious Hepatitis" because you can get easily infected by the Hep A virus through contaminated food, water and personal contact. The serologic analysis of the presence of the Hepatitis A virus (HAV) in infected persons serves as a conclusive diagnosis of the condition.

Hepatitis

Hepatitis B is also called "serum Hepatitis". The Hepatitis B virus (HBV) can be transmitted through sexual intercourse, parenteral route (intravenous or injection), and perinatal (through the placenta by the mother). Just like Hepatitis A, the serologic analysis of the presence of the Hep B virus in infected persons serves as a conclusive diagnosis of the condition.

Hepatitis C

Hepatitis C virus (HCV), the infecting agent of Hepatitis C, can be transmitted primarily through blood transfusions. Less frequently, you can also acquire it through sexual activities, fecal contamination of food, ingestion of contaminated food and water and through parenteral routes. This means that you can acquire the infection through any open wound in your body that is exposed to the virus. Sharing contaminated needles has been one of the most common transmission routes for Hepatitis C. This is the reason why drug users are potentially at greater risk of infection.

Hepatitis D

It's also called delta Hepatitis. The Hepatitis D virus (HDV) infects only those who have Hepatitis B. It's unique in this sense because it doesn't infect individuals who don't have Hepatitis B.

Hepatitis E

This type of Hepatitis is caused by the Hep E virus (HEV), and is transmitted through the fecal-oral route. If you're infected with the HEV and you don't wash your hands properly when you defecate, you can infect other people.

All these viruses, HAV, HBV, HCV, HDV and HEV, attack the nucleus of the cells of your liver causing inflammation. Since this book is about Hepatitis C, let's focus more on this type of Hepatitis.

Hepatitis C history

Previously, Hepatitis C was classified as either Hepatitis A or Hepatitis B. But later on, it was discovered that it is distinct from A and B. It was discovered that the HCV can be found in the Ribonucleic Acid (RNA) of the cell. This makes it different from the rest of the Hepatitis viruses, which are typically found in the Deoxyribonucleic Acid (DNA) of the cell.

It has been established too that 3% of blood donors in the US are HCV positive; hence there is a need to test the blood for the virus before any transfusion is performed. Likewise, detection of the HCV is crucial to prevent serious liver illnesses developing later on. The liver is the major organ that metabolizes food, detoxifies and synthesizes essential substances needed by the body. Any damage to the liver can impair your health significantly.

Hep C carriers

People can have Hepatitis C without showing any symptoms, especially during the first few months of the disorder. They are called "carriers" because they can carry the infecting virus, but they don't get sick. However, a positive result should always merit treatment. This is to avoid the disorder worsening to carcinoma (cancer), cirrhosis and chronic Hepatitis that can cause death.

Food handlers must always be tested for the Hepatitis viruses to prevent transmitting the infection to unsuspecting individuals.

How to detect a Hepatitis C infection

Hep C can rarely be detected during the first few months of the infection. It can only be detected during the latent stages by serologic screening tests, and confirmatory tests to prove the existence of the

HCV. Having an annual test for the presence of the virus is advisable in areas where the viral infection is prevalent.

There are convenient screening card tests that can be performed within 30 minutes. You can actually perform them at home. But be sure to wear gloves and protective gear. You must also follow the simple instructions that accompany the card or test kit accurately. If the screening test is positive, a confirmatory test must be done by a licensed laboratory to confirm the results. This will eliminate false positive results. Once the confirmatory test is positive, appropriate treatment must commence.

Chapter 2: Cause and Symptoms of Hepatitis C

The cause of the Hepatitis C infection is the Hepatitis C virus or HCV. Once the virus enters your body, it stays in your RNA and destroys your cells. The primary organ affected is your liver, which is the major metabolic organ. Your liver has a crucial role in keeping you healthy and fit, and any injury to its cells will cause illnesses.

Symptoms of Hepatitis C

There are varying symptoms of the Hepatitis C infection. Some individuals may not even display the symptoms. They are called asymptomatic carriers. But if you're experiencing any of these symptoms, you have to consult your doctor immediately:

- Fatigue
- Nausea and vomiting
- Weakness
- Fever
- Bruising
- Swollen stomach
- Loss of appetite
- Muscle weakness

- Swollen ankles
- Stomach pains

In extreme cases, the person may also experience:

- Dark colored urine—Usually tea colored, or deep yellow
- Jaundice—Yellowing of the skin, the sclera of the eyes and of the mucus membranes
- Light colored stool

These symptoms may occur simultaneously or gradually. You have to be alert when you notice any of these symptoms appearing in any individual, so you can consult your doctor ASAP.

There may be symptoms in some individuals that are not mentioned here because of individual differences. You will have to be on the lookout for one or two symptoms using these lists. If you have checked more than one of these symptoms, it's an indication that it's time you should visit your doctor. Don't ignore these warning signals. Early treatment can increase a good prognosis of Hepatitis infected patients.

Chapter 3: How to Treat Hepatitis C

Viruses cannot be killed by drugs, but their symptoms can be treated using medications, and their progress can be deterred. You have to know about the medications used in treating Hepatitis, so you can manage Hepatitis C effectively. Take note that treatment usually lasts from 3 months to 1 year, or extended accordingly. Here are some medications employed for Hepatitis C.

1. **Interferon (IFN) plus ribavirin**

    This is also called the dual therapy because it combines interferon and ribavirin. Both of these drugs are needed to prevent the viral infection from worsening. The interferon will destroy the RNA that hosts the virus to inhibit viral activity. Aside from having anti-inflammatory actions, interferon also helps the immune system in its defense against these infecting agents.

    On the other hand, ribavirin is believed to inhibit viral replication. More studies are being conducted for the specific action of ribavirin on Hepatitis viruses, A, B, C, D, and E.

Side effects of interferon and ribavirin

- Increased risk of myocardial infarction (heart attack)
- Nausea
- Hemolytic anemia
- Muscle pains
- Vomiting
- Loss of appetite
- Flu-like symptoms
- Blood disorders (thrombocytopenia—low platelet count; neutropenia—low neutrophil count)
- Hair loss
- Headache

The serious side effect is that it can cause lung problems that can lead to death.

2. Interferon plus ribavirin and telaprevir (simeprevir or boceprevir)

This has been recently approved by the Food and Drug Administration (FDA), especially for individuals who are genotype 1. It has been observed that the addition of telaprevir increases the chances of the treatment. Telaprevir helps ribavirin in inhibiting the multiplication of the Hep C virus, and together they act to prevent the reproduction of the virus in the body cells.

Side effects of telaprevir

- Headache
- Anemia
- Diarrhea
- Hemorrhoids
- Lowers white blood cells (WBC)
- Itching

3. Sofosbuvir plus simeprevir

This has been recently discovered and is in its phase 2 study. It has 90% proven effectiveness against the Hep C virus among a group of patients. There were reported minor side effects, such as rash and sunburn.

4. Liver supplement

Essentiale contains essential phospholipids which can replace the degenerated phospholipids in your liver cells. This will promote the growth of new Hepatic cells.

Side effects of Essentiale

- Diarrhea
- Severe allergy in some persons
- Stomachache
- Nausea

5. Liver transplant

The liver has important functions in the body and if it is not functioning well, the body becomes poisoned and the whole metabolism impaired. This will affect all the bodily processes and prevent the normal functioning of organs. Therefore, when the liver shuts down completely the body needs a new liver to restore proper function, and a liver transplant is the last resort.

These are the medical treatments used for Hep C. Take note that there are harmful side effects of these therapeutic drugs, as well. Use these drugs only upon the prescription of a health specialist or a doctor

Chapter 4: Home Prevention and Treatment

There are effective and simple prevention and treatment methods that you can use at home for Hepatitis C disorders in conjunction with your prescribed medication. The most important thing to remember is to prevent the infection from occurring. This is a safer way to stay healthy than trying to cure what is incurable. Knowing how to do this will help significantly in managing the condition.

Home Prevention

1. **Rest more**

    Acute viral infections are generally self-limiting; they go away by themselves after a certain period of time. But with Hep C, the virus infection is usually chronic, so it stays in the body longer. That's why you need more rest to allow your immune system to recover quickly and prevent the spread of the infection. This is an important technique that you must remember. You have to rest, rest and rest so you can get well quickly. Most especially prohibited is lifting weights. This can exert undue pressure on your liver further stressing it out aggravating the disorder.

2. Avoid fatty foods

Fatty foods tend to accumulate in your Hepatic cells causing fatty liver. This condition can worsen and affect the total function of your liver. In the presence of HCV, there's no escape for your liver, it will definitely be damaged. Junk those meat fats and creamy foods because they aid in the destruction of your liver cells.

3. Derive your sweets from fruits and honey

It has been demonstrated that natural sweets such as, fruits and honey tend to boost your liver function and immune system.

4. Maintain a healthy weight

Maintaining a healthy weight helps to boost your immune response and keep you healthy. When you're healthy you're less likely to get infected with the Hep C virus.

5. **Eat a balanced diet**

   A balanced diet will also help to maintain your health and lessen the risk of you contracting an infection. A balanced diet is composed of 50% carbohydrates (rice, pasta, bread); 20% fats (dairy products, vegetable fats); 20% protein (fish, lean meat, peas); and 10% vitamins (A, B, C, D, E) from fruits, vegetables and sunlight.

6. **Exercise regularly**

   By exercising regularly, you're enhancing your immune system, thereby, lessening your propensity in acquiring the viral infection. A 30-minute to 1 hour exercise daily is recommended. Exercise does not only shed your excess fats but it also induces whole body relaxation, especially after the exercise.

7. **Avoid alcohol**

   Alcohol has a detrimental effect on the liver because of the action of its metabolites in killing Hepatic or liver cells. Acetaldehyde, the end product of alcohol metabolism causes the hardening or necrosis of the Hepatic cells. With alcoholism, the liver cells will slowly die until liver necrosis occurs. This will now lead to liver failure and eventual death.

8. Avoid any substance that stresses the liver and kidneys

Anything that enters your body adds extra load to your major metabolic organ—your liver, and your major excretory organ—your kidneys. There are some substances that exert undue workload such as, analgesics, caffeine, refined sugar, chocolates, black teas, table salt, aspirin and ibuprofen. These substances must be avoided or should be taken in moderation because they tend to have detrimental effects on your liver.

9. Eat more fruits, vegetables and nuts

The anti-oxidant and antimicrobial properties of fruits, vegetables and nuts, and the essential vitamins and substances derived from them help a lot in the control of the viral infection. Hence, eat more of these foodstuffs.

Home Treatment

1. **Natural honey**

   This can be taken one teaspoon thrice a day, or mixed with drinks and beverages. It acts as a vitamin for the liver to hasten healing of cells.

2. **Milk thistle**

   The active component of milk thistle, which is silymarin helps in the growth and development of new cells to replace the cells damaged by the Hep C virus. It also inhibits the growth of the Hep C virus, preventing its multiplication.

   Recent studies showed that when silymarin is combined with interferon, it produces excellent results in treating Hepatitis C infections. Also, silymarin in combination with alpha lipoic acid and selenium was proven as an effective trio to treat Hepatitis C.

3. Licorice root

Licorice root has an active component, glycyrrhizin that can help prevent cancer or carcinoma. It can be used as a substitute for milk thistle to inhibit the growth of the HCV.

4. Flaxseed oil

Flaxseed oil helps prevent the growth of the Hep C virus. It also acts as a supplement to maintain your health and well-being. Its component alpha-linolenic acid aids in the treatment of inflammation. You can combine it with non- homogenized yogurt to enhance its effectiveness.

5. Vitamin C

Large doses of vitamin C can be taken in to help in the elimination of viral symptoms, and delay growth of the virus. The immune system is believed to be enhanced by vitamin C. Vitamin C can not only readily be found in citrus fruits such as lemon and oranges, but also in guavas and mangoes.

6. Sunlight

Sunlight helps produce vitamin D, which acts to strengthen the body from viral infections. Expose yourself to the harmless early morning rays of the sun.

These are the home prevention and treatment techniques for Hepatitis C that you can use appropriately.

Chapter 5: Complementary Treatments for Hepatitis C

These complementary treatments for Hepatitis C infection are still under study and *there are no intensive clinical trials to prove their effectiveness.* Nevertheless, these methods are believed to have helped in reducing the symptoms of Hep C. These complementary methods are not used on their own but in conjunction with other medical treatments. These adjunctive treatments must also be approved by your attending physician before you start implementing them.

1. **Acupuncture**

    Acupuncture is a method that makes use of needles to apply pressure on certain meridian points in your body that are connected to specific body parts. The Chinese believed that everything produces energy; that the body has also a Chi (energy force) that should flow smoothly for a person to stay healthy.

    In acupuncture, the application of needles in these meridian points will help restore the balance of the body's energy and cure the body of illnesses. Acupuncture acts in removing blockages in this energy flow between the Yin (positive) and Yang (negative) energies. When a balanced Chi is achieved, this helps the person get well.

While acupuncture can be used with your doctor's permission, reflexology is not recommended because of the danger of inflicting further side effects in infectious diseases.

For acupuncture, it has been observed to have reduced headaches, muscle aches, fatigue and the other symptoms of Hep C infection. It can also aid in the relaxation of your body just like massage therapy, and can contribute to the maintenance of liver health by preventing the spread of the inflammation.

Acupuncture is utilized alongside medical treatments to facilitate treatment and recuperation.

Contraindications

Contraindications for the use of acupuncture as adjunct treatment for Hepatitis C infection are the following:

- Hepatitis B infection
- Hematologic diseases
- Uncontrolled diabetes
- Alcoholic liver disease
- Liver cancer
- Anemia
- HIV infection
- Psychiatric condition
- Recent surgical procedure

When a person has these conditions, acupuncture could not be used as a complementary treatment for Hepatitis C infections.

2. Massage therapy

There are various massage techniques that you can use to help treat Hep C. The rolling, friction, vibration, kneading, tapotement, and finger-walking massages can be done using the fingers, thumb, elbows and palms. Direct massage of the liver is not advisable though. The legs and arms can be massaged gently to enhance circulation and muscle strength in the musculoskeletal and circulatory systems.

The purpose of the massage is to relax the muscles and to promote proper circulation so that sufficient nourishment and oxygen can reach the cells in different parts of the body. These cells can perform their functions effectively when they're healthy. If the Hep C condition is already cancerous, massage is not advisable because this may worsen the condition.

Contraindications

- o Cancer
- o HIV infection
- o Hematologic disease
- o Open wounds
- o Recent surgical procedure

Precautions

In both acupuncture and massage techniques, it's advisable for the person performing the technique to use gloves if he has open wounds. This is to prevent infecting himself with the virus. Remember that you're dealing with an infectious virus.

After treatment, used materials such as needles and blood contaminated items must be disposed of properly to trash cans for infectious items. Materials must be decontaminated properly through sterilization. If there are no potential sources of infection, the personal paraphernalia (blankets, beddings, and clothing) of the infected person must be regularly changed and sterilized or boiled. Although viruses are not killed through high temperatures, other microorganisms can be eliminated through heat. Avoid the spread of infection by observing personal hygiene and hygienic practices.

3. **Meditation and visualization**

   Meditation and visualization can help in your rest and relaxation. Studies have proven that meditation can provide rest and relaxation, which you need when you're sick with Hepatitis C. On the other hand visualization can help establish a positive mental conditioning that will increase your chances of a better prognosis. If you believe you can cope with the condition, then this will help you significantly in overcoming the infection.

4. Ayurvedic

This method originated from India and has been used by some health practitioners in the West. It's similar to the TCM (Traditional Chinese Medicine) of China because it uses herbs. Ayurvedic herbs such as, guduchi, andrographis paniculata and haritaki are used in treating Hep C. Keep in mind though, that ayurvedic is not for all individuals. Just because these are herbs doesn't mean that you can use them randomly, either. Your doctor still has the final say on what you can ingest and on what you can adopt as a complementary treatment. What's important is that you know about these herbs.

Guduchi

Also known as heart-leave moonseed, this herb contains a phytochemical, berberine that is used in treating liver Hepatitis and Jaundice. It helps in preventing the growth of liver cancer cells and enhances the function of the immune system. It can serve as a liver tonic and is useful in digestive problems too. All the parts of the herb can be used by converting it into juice form through decocting the herb. But it is the stem that is most useful. The stem can be grinded or crushed with water to come up with the juice. This can be taken orally twice or thrice a day.

Andrographis paniculata

This herb contains a phytochemical, too, identified as andrographolides. This active component has been observed to boost the immune system. It prevents the spread of inflammation and protects the Hepatic cells. It has reported healing effects too on HIV infections, Hepatitis, Syphilis, Jaundice, Upper Respiratory problems and many other infectious diseases. The leaf and underground stem can be taken orally or used topically. It can also be turned into a powder or a tablet for easy ingestion and taken twice or thrice daily.

Haritaki

Also known as Chebulic myrobalan, this fruit herb helps in the treatment of Hep C by rejuvenating cells and tissues. It also has anti-anxiety properties and promotes digestion and metabolism of foodstuffs. It can be ingested by dissolving the haritaki powder in water or as prescribed by the Ayurvedic doctor. You can take it in divided doses, twice or thrice daily.

Contraindications

- Pregnant women—It is contraindicated because it can be harmful to the baby
- Allergy—Allergy to any of the components of the herbs can be fatal
- Thin or underweight people
- Menstrual periods—Before, during and after the period
- Breast feeding mothers
- Tired or fatigued persons
- Diabetes mellitus
- Weakened individuals
- Severe dehydration
- Kava and comfrey—These are herbs that are contraindicated in Hep C because they damage the liver instead of boosting its function

5. Aromatherapy

This method makes use the aroma of certain plants and herbs to relieve stress and anxiety. The lavender oil is the most common oil used in baths, massages or inhalants to soothe the nerves and to induce a relaxed mood. It has been reported that patients using aromatherapy have better healing chances.

Contraindications

- Allergy to lavender oil or to the plant used
- Pregnant mothers, unless recommended by obstetrician

These complementary methods are slowly undergoing more intensive and extensive trials and studies to firmly establish their significance in the treatment of Hepatitis C.

Chapter 6: Complications of Hepatitis C

As previously mentioned, untreated Hepatitis C infection can result to liver cirrhosis, carcinoma (cancer) or chronic Hepatitis. These are all serious conditions that can cause death, If not treated promptly. Aside from these, here are other complications of Hepatitis C disorder.

1. **Jaundice**

    This condition is characterized by a yellowish discoloration of the skin, the mucus membranes and the sclera of the eyes. It's caused by the insufficient elimination and conjugation of bilirubin by the liver. The liver is responsible in rendering bilirubin in a soluble form so it can easily be excreted from the body. When the liver can no longer perform its metabolic and detoxification functions, jaundice results. The urine will also acquire an amber or tea color. So, if you have this disease, you'll be yellow skinned. If your skin starts to turn yellow, don't hesitate to consult your doctor before it gets too late.

2. Brain damage

The liver is impaired when there's Hepatitis C infection. When the liver is impaired, it cannot convert ammonia to its soluble form, so it cannot be excreted properly. Ammonia is one of the waste products of biological processes in the body. When ammonia accumulates in your bloodstream, it causes toxicity primarily in your brain and central nervous system. This can result to brain damage, coma and eventual death.

3. Hemorrhage

The liver is also the organ that synthesizes clotting factors needed in blood clotting. When the liver cannot produce these clotting factors in sufficient amounts, the body cannot clot blood properly so that hemorrhaging occurs. Bruising and hematoma can occur easily too. This can prove deadly when there are big wounds and bleeding doesn't stop. The person will bleed to death.

4. Underdevelopment of sexual characteristics

The liver is also responsible in producing cholesterol, which is the basic structure of all steroid hormones. The steroid hormones include your testosterone and estrogen, which are your major female and male sexual hormones. When the liver is dysfunctional, cholesterol is produced insufficiently thereby creating steroid hormones that are underdeveloped too. This leads to underdeveloped secondary male and female sexual characteristics such as, high pitched voice, and growth of breasts in males. In females, hirsutism (facial hair), and underdeveloped breasts will occur.

5. **Ascites**

This is the accumulation of fluid in the liver that can affect the abdominal cavity. This can result to a more serious disease called peritonitis. Peritonitis is the infection of the accumulated fluid by invading pathologic microorganisms.

6. **Liver failure**

Liver shutdown or failure can occur if treatment is not initiated immediately. When this happens, the only solution is a liver transplant. At this stage, all the Hepatic cells are keratinized and are no longer functioning.

These are the complications that you have to prevent by treating your Hepatitis C promptly. Don't ignore any symptoms that manifest outwardly. Consult your doctor immediately so that diagnostic and laboratory tests can be performed to determine your illness.

Chapter 7: Valuable Pointers about Hepatitis C

Hepatitis C is only one type of the Hepatitis infection, but it's a silent killer. Hence, you have to beware of it. It might be creeping into your system slowly and you still don't know it. All the information presented in this book will assist you in being watchful. In addition, here are some valuable pointers about Hepatitis C treatment that you must know.

1. **Beware of blood transfusions.** The primary route of acquiring Hep C is through blood so be cautious in accepting blood from other people. Blood banks have made it a point to test for the Hep C before blood donations, but some third world countries are still lacking in appropriate lab materials. Allow yourself to be transfused only when it's a matter of life and death. In this manner, you can also avoid HIV infections.

2. **Avoid sexual promiscuity.** Although, sexual contact is not the common route of acquiring the HCV, don't get intimate just with anyone. This is where being monogamous is advantageous. Kissing is a low risk method too of acquiring the virus because they're not

present in large amounts in your mouth. BUT if you have lesions or blisters in your sex organs and in your mouth, then this will increase your risk of acquiring the infection.

3. **There is no vaccination against Hepatitis C.** Hepatitis A and Hepatitis B have a common vaccine but not Hep C. This is because Hep C has several genotypes and there are no viable animal cell culture models. Remember to immunize your child against Hepatitis A and B.

4. **Condoms don't ensure 100% protection against Hep C infection.** Condoms can tear and allow the virus to seep inside your wounds or open skin. The mucus membranes that line the sexual organs are typically sensitive and can be easily damaged.

5. **Watch out for contaminated razors.** Razor blades contaminated with Hep C can cause infection. This goes with nail cutters too. The infected person should have a razor blade and a nail cutter for himself only because open wounds when shaving and cutting your nails are common ways to get infected with the virus.

6. **Any drug can subject the liver to undue load.** Anything that enters your body generally passes through your liver, because the liver is the "first-pass route". Even therapeutic drugs will add more load to your liver that can tax your cells. Therefore, take in only medications when extremely needed.

7. **Use only liver supplements that are officially approved.** There are numerous liver supplements offered online and all are claiming miraculous cures. If it sounds too good to be true, it is! Buy only those supplements that have the FDA (Food and Drug Administration) stamp of approval, or the National Center for Complementary and Alternative Medicine's recommendation.

8. **Wash your hands often.** Hand-washing is still one of the most effective ways to prevent infection. So, wash your hands every time you can, especially before and after eating.

9. **Hepatitis C infection is most prevalent in third world countries.** Hence, take extra precautions when visiting third world countries. Use the information on prevention presented in this book to avoid infecting yourself.

10. **Hepatitis C can infect anyone.** Your age, gender and nationality don't matter. Once the virus enters your body, you will surely get infected. But a healthy lifestyle will decrease your risk of contracting the disease.

11. **You can use yoga as a meditation method.** You can use any technique as long as this can induce rest and relaxation. You need rest to fight the Hep C infection.

12. **The secret is to use protective gear when you have open wounds.** Getting close to a person with the Hep C virus doesn't necessarily get you infected, unless you are transfused with his blood, or you have open wounds or skin incisions where the virus can penetrate and enter.

Learn all these valuable pointers so that you will know when to protect yourself and when not to worry. You can combine your knowledge of these pointers and the information in the previous chapters to prevent acquiring the Hepatitis C infection.

Conclusion

The Hep C treatment methods described in this book are proven to have alleviated the symptoms of the infection and have prevented fatal complications. Get acquainted with them so you will have an idea of their actions and contraindications.

However, keep in mind that prevention is always better than cure, so strive to prevent this virus from infecting you or your loved ones. Implement the prevention techniques in your household immediately. These home prevention methods will also reduce the threat of other infectious diseases from wreaking havoc in the healthy atmosphere of your home.

Finally, I'd like to thank you for purchasing this book! If you found it helpful, I'd greatly appreciate it if you'd take a moment to leave a review on Amazon. Thank you!

Made in United States
North Haven, CT
15 October 2023

42775834R00033